STRATEGIC PLAN
DIVISION OF HIV/AIDS PREVENTION
2011 THROUGH 2015

National Center for HIV/AIDS, Viral Hepatitis, STD, and TB Prevention
Division of HIV/AIDS Prevention

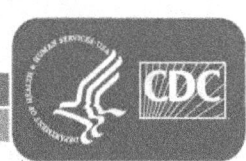

STRATEGIC PLAN
DIVISION OF HIV/AIDS PREVENTION
2011 THROUGH 2015

U.S. Department of Health and Human Services
Centers for Disease Control and Prevention
National Center for HIV/AIDS, Viral Hepatitis, STD, and TB Prevention
August 2011

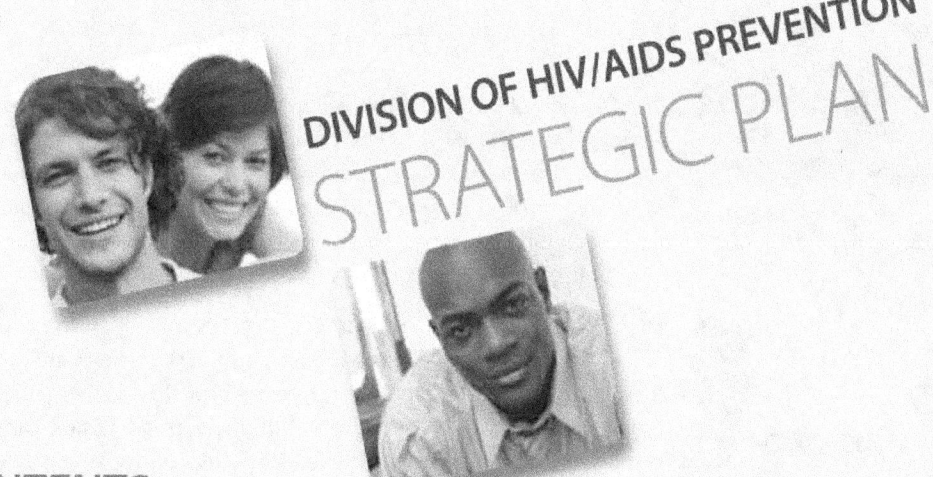

DIVISION OF HIV/AIDS PREVENTION

STRATEGIC PLAN

CONTENTS

Message from the Director 2

Introduction 4

The Plan 10

Next Steps 24

Appendix A — List of Acronyms 25

Appendix B — Goals, Objectives, and Strategies 26

Appendix C — Links to NHAS and NCHHSTP Plans 30

Appendix D — Goals and Objectives, with Baselines, Targets, and Data Source 34

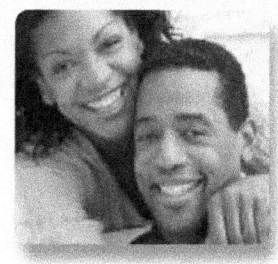

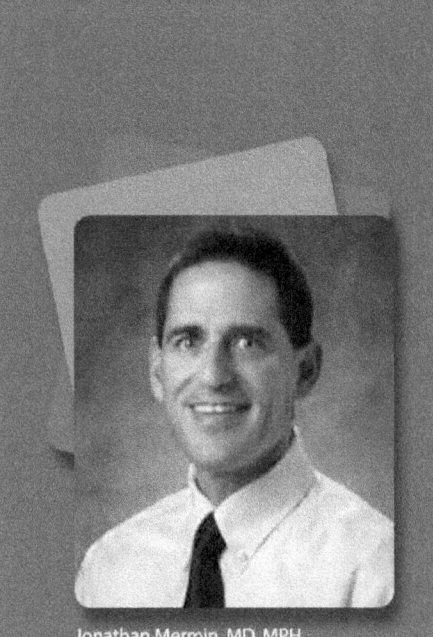

Jonathan Mermin, MD, MPH

The Plan reflects the Division's response to new opportunities and imperatives for HIV prevention created by critical shifts in the national, state, and local economic and policy environments

Message from the Director

The Division of HIV/AIDS Prevention (DHAP) is pleased to present its Strategic Plan 2011-2015 (hereafter, the Plan). The Plan encompasses all aspects of the Division's work and will serve as a practical guide to inform development of work plans to ensure DHAP activities and resources are aligned with its priorities. This Plan is DHAP's blueprint for achieving its vision of a future free of HIV. We are committed to its implementation.

DHAP's Plan is the result of a process that began with an External Peer Review of DHAP Surveillance, Research, and HIV Prevention Programs held in April 2009. This multi-day meeting brought together more than 70 experts, including scientists, state health directors, advocates, partners, and community members, to provide feedback and guidance on DHAP scientific and programmatic activities. In the months that followed, more than 80 CDC staff—both internal and external to the Division—engaged in discussions, planning sessions, and two 2-day retreats, including a final, follow-up session, focused on the most efficient and effective path to ensuring reductions in HIV incidence and disparities. At several points along the way, all DHAP staff—more than 700 people—were offered the opportunity to provide input, including participation in an organization-wide survey (November 2010) to submit comments on the proposed goals, objectives, and strategies found in Appendix B.

As the planning process evolved, DHAP's external partners remained engaged. In early 2010, 30 partners were interviewed, providing their thoughts on a variety of issues including areas DHAP should focus on, external factors that would influence success, and opportunities for partnering. In addition, members of the External Peer Review steering committee were invited to participate on a Strategic Plan External Work Group and comment on the components of the Plan, culminating in an in-person meeting in November 2010 to review a draft copy.

As a result of this expansive process, the Plan reflects the Division's response to new opportunities and imperatives for HIV prevention created by critical shifts in the national, state, and local economic and policy environments, including the passage of health care legislation and the July 2010 release of the National HIV/AIDS Strategy for the United States (NHAS). The Plan emphasizes maximizing our effect on the epidemic and internal and external coordination and collaboration, calling for accountability at every level, strategic allocation of resources, and the development and use of objective planning and transparent decision-making frameworks across DHAP's HIV prevention portfolio. The Plan also underscores the important role of partnerships in both reducing HIV incidence and addressing the disparities that persist among populations and within communities.

Already, the Plan is making a difference in how the Division operates. For example:

- In keeping with the NHAS priority of targeting federal HIV prevention funding to jurisdictions with the greatest need, DHAP developed a new algorithm for its cooperative agreements that fund health departments. The new funding announcements emphasize maximizing the effect of interventions and strategies to achieve the highest return on investment.

- Through collaborations with other HHS agencies including the Health Resources and Services Administration and Indian Health Service, and inter-agency funding agreements with the National Institutes of Health, DHAP is helping to leverage limited resources to fund new research to increase the effectiveness of federal HIV prevention activities.

- DHAP has implemented efforts to streamline grantee reporting requirements and increase transparency in how and why decisions are made.

- As part of the Enhanced Comprehensive HIV Prevention Planning (ECHPP) project, DHAP is supporting implementation and monitoring of plans developed by the 12 jurisdictions with the greatest burden of AIDS (based on 2007 data). These plans focus on coordinating prevention activities to identify and address gaps in scope and reach of prevention interventions and strategies among high-risk populations. This project is a component of a wider multi-agency effort coordinated by the U.S. Department of Health and Human Services (HHS).

- DHAP has increased efforts to model prevention efforts in the U.S. and local jurisdiction, and optimize cost-effectiveness and impact.

- DHAP is funding 65 jurisdictions to enhance laboratory reporting of CD4 and viral load data. Measuring community viral load (CVL) and other care indicators allows cities to gauge effectiveness of efforts to improve the health of people living with HIV.

- DHAP recently established an Office of Health Equity which provides leadership on understanding the determinants of and strategies for addressing HIV and AIDS inequities, and coordinates and monitors the Division's activities related to reducing health inequities among populations and risk groups disproportionately affected by the epidemic.

Over the next 6 months, all DHAP branches and operating units will update work plans to map current activities to the Plan. These work plans will identify specific deliverables, the team or individual responsible, and the timeframe for completion. This information will allow DHAP leaders to ensure project alignment with the priorities identified during Plan implementation, guiding decision making about what activities DHAP should limit, what it should be doing more of, and what new activities it should undertake.

DHAP appreciates the ideas, suggestions, and expertise contributed by CDC staff to the creation of the Plan. And we appreciate the partners who participated in the April 2009 External Peer Review for providing extensive comments and suggestions and to those partners who continued to participate as members of the Strategic Plan External Work Group. I am honored to work with you and look forward to achieving our mission of preventing HIV infection and reducing the incidence of HIV-related illness and death, in collaboration with community, state, national and international partners.

Jonathan Mermin, MD, MPH
Director, Division of HIV/AIDS Prevention, NCHHSTP
Centers for Disease Control and Prevention

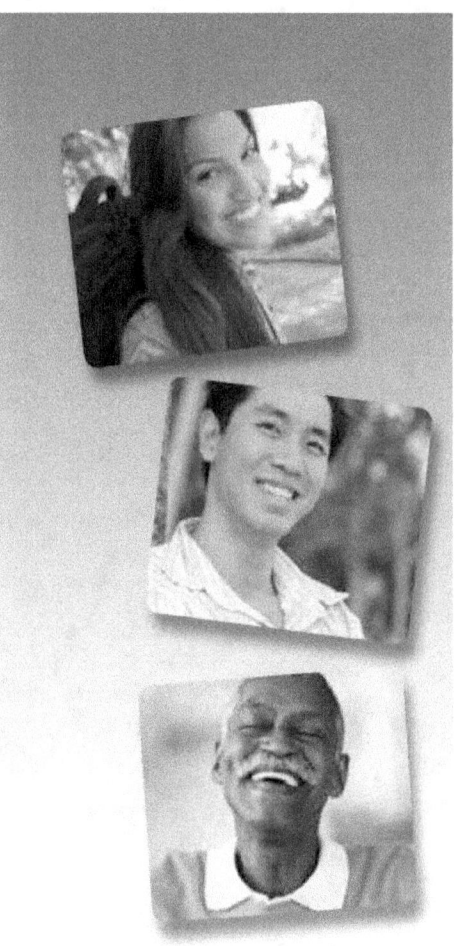

Introduction

The HIV epidemic in the United States impacts the lives of hundreds of thousands of individuals every day, a fact underscored by the release of the first National HIV/AIDS Strategy for the nation in July 2010. The latest estimates from the Centers for Disease Control and Prevention (CDC) suggest about 50,000 people become infected with HIV each year,[1] and that 1.2 million people in this country are now living with HIV.[2] Of those 1.2 million, an estimated 20.1% are unaware of their infections.[3]

Analysis of surveillance data also reveals tremendous disparities in HIV among populations: African Americans are eight times more likely to be living with HIV than whites and Hispanics/Latinos are three times more likely than whites.[4] In addition, the rate of new HIV diagnoses among men of all races and ethnicities who have sex with other men (MSM) is more than 44 times that of other men and more than 40 times that of women.[5] Marked differences also exist in the geographic distribution of AIDS cases in the United States: 50 percent of people living with AIDS reside in only five states, while 90 percent of persons living with AIDS reside in 23 states.[6]

DHAP's Guiding Principles:

We believe...

- Effective leadership requires clear vision, insight, and effective communication.
- The need for innovative solutions requires us to encourage creativity, intellectual curiosity and openness to change.
- That because the quality of our work is determined by the character of our staff, we must uphold high standards of conduct including integrity, respect, and dedication.
- That a positive, productive, and enjoyable workplace requires staff have positive attitudes.

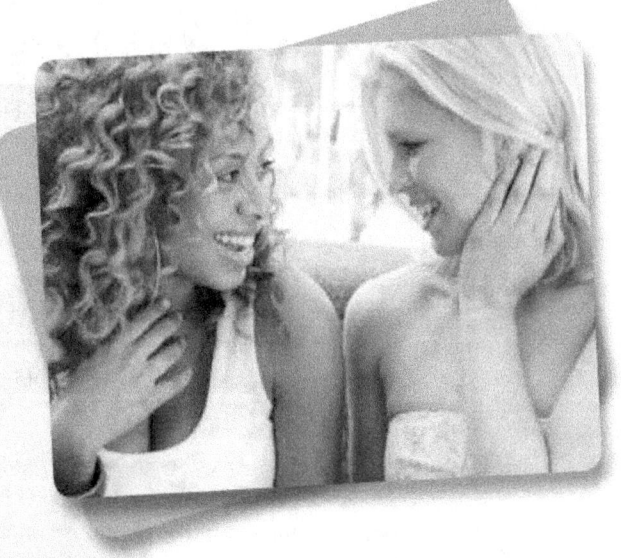

[1] Prejean J, Song R, Hernandez A, Ziebell R, Green T, et al. (2011) Estimated HIV Incidence in the United States, 2006–2009. PLoS ONE 6(8): e17502. doi:10.1371/journal.pone.0017502 www.plosone.org/article/info%3Adoi%2F10.1371%2Fjournal.pone.0017502

[2] CDC. HIV Surveillance—United States,1981-2008. MMWR 2011;60(21):659-93; available at www.cdc.gov/mmwr/preview/mmwrhtml/mm6021a2.htm?s_cid=mm6021a2_w

[3] Ibid.

[4] CDC, HIV Surveillance Report,2009 available at ww.cdc.gov/hiv/surveillance/resources/reports

[5] Abstract: Calculating HIV and Syphilis Rates for Risk Groups: Estimating the National Population Size of Men Who Have Sex with Men, DW Purcell, C Johnson, A Lansky, J Prejean, R Stein, P Denning, Z Gaul, H Weinstock, J Su, & N Crepaz, Latebreaker #22896 Presented March 10, 2010, 2010 National STD Prevention Conference; Atlanta, GA.

[6] CDC, HIV Surveillance Report, 2008. Published June 2010; available at www.cdc.gov/hiv/surveillance/resources/reports

HIV Prevention Works

Despite the significant challenges highlighted by these data, HIV in this country is not inevitable. Over the last 3 decades, the HIV prevention community has developed a portfolio of proven strategies that can be deployed to reduce the risk of acquiring or transmitting HIV, including: HIV testing; evidence-based interventions for people living with HIV or at high risk for HIV; partner services; antiretroviral therapy; substance abuse treatment; access to condoms and sterile syringes; and screening and treatment for other sexually transmitted infections.

The key to achieving a future free of HIV is using what we have learned about implementing these proven strategies to ensure the most effective combination of approaches, from both a programmatic and cost perspective, are targeted to the populations most at risk and brought to scale—an approach referred to throughout this document as "high impact prevention." This requires prioritizing the allocation of prevention resources, careful monitoring and constant re-evaluation, targeted research, and intensive and sustained collaboration and coordination with partners.

Prevention Success by the Numbers

- Since the mid-1980s, the HIV transmission rate—the estimated annual number of new HIV infections per 100 persons living with HIV—declined approximately 89% (from 44 transmissions per 100 people in 1984 to 5 transmissions per 100 people in 2006).[1]
- Perinatal HIV infections—those transmitted from mother to child—have decreased from 1,000-2,000 per year in the early 1990s to an estimated 138 per year in 2004.[2]
- The proportion of persons who know they are infected with HIV increased from 75% in 2003 to 79% in 2006.[3]
- For every HIV infection that is prevented, an estimated $355,000 (in 2008 dollars) is saved in the cost of providing lifetime HIV treatment.[4]

[1] Holtgrave DR, Hall HI, Rhodes PH, et al. Updated annual HIV transmission rates in the United States, 1977 2006. J Acquir Immune Defic Syndr 2009;50(2):236 238.

[2] McKenna M, Hu X. Recent trends in the incidence and morbidity that are associated with perinatal human immunodeficiency virus infection in the United States. Am J Obstet and Gynecol, 2007; 197(3), Suppl: S10 S16.

[3] CDC. HIV prevalence estimates – United States, 2006. MMWR 2008;57(39):1073 1076.

[4] Schackman BR, Gebo KA, Walensky RP, et al. The lifetime cost of current human immunodeficiency virus care in the United States. Med Care 2006 Nov;44(11):990 997

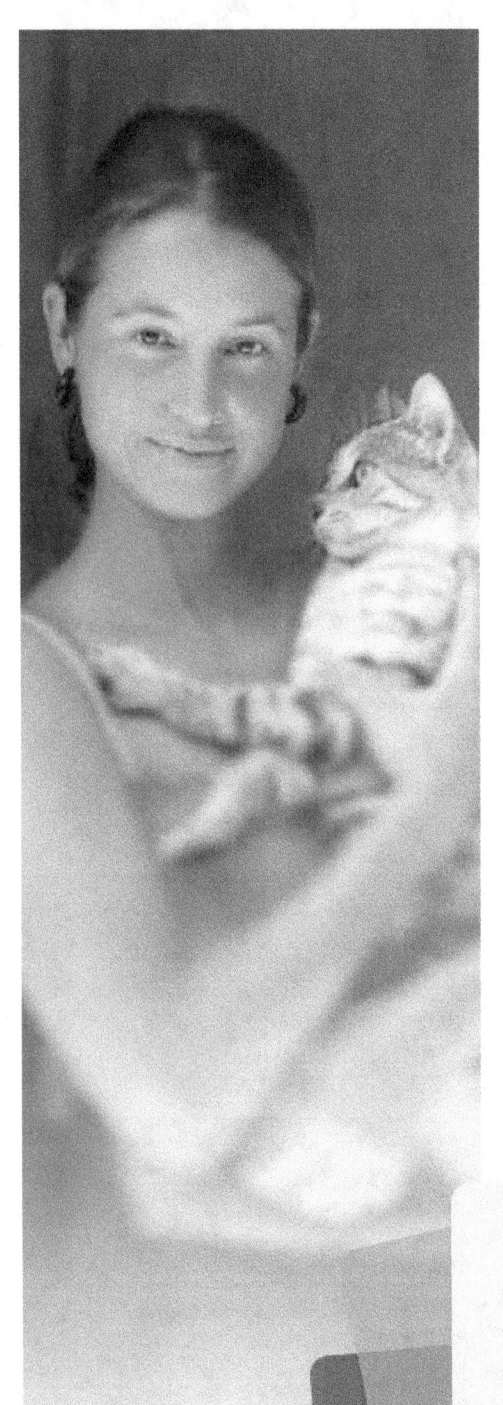

CDC's Division of HIV/AIDS Prevention

Since the very beginning of the epidemic, CDC has often been at the forefront of efforts to prevent the spread of HIV. While not representing all aspects of the agency's response, CDC's Division of HIV/AIDS Prevention (DHAP), located in the National Center for HIV/AIDS, Viral Hepatitis, STD, and TB Prevention (NCHHSTP), oversees the majority of CDC's domestic HIV prevention activities. The Division provides national leadership and support for surveillance, prevention research and programs, and the development, implementation, and evaluation of evidence-based interventions serving populations affected by or at risk of HIV infection.

Given this critical role in domestic HIV prevention, DHAP's top priority is to strategically allocate its surveillance, research, and programmatic funding to produce the greatest impact on the epidemic. This obligation has taken on even greater importance in recent years due to economic challenges experienced by HIV prevention programs at the state and local level. At the same time, there are also several new opportunities for improving the impact of HIV prevention programs. First, national interest in health care has increased opportunities to evaluate new models for seamlessly linking and integrating prevention and care. Second, advances in prevention science, as well as the ability to more precisely map and track the epidemic, have resulted in new opportunities to reduce incidence. Finally, the publication of the first National HIV/AIDS Strategy in July 2010 created new opportunities for advancing high-impact prevention.

Division of HIV/AIDS Prevention

Vision: A future free of HIV

Mission: To promote health and quality of life by preventing HIV infection and reducing HIV-related illness and death in the United States

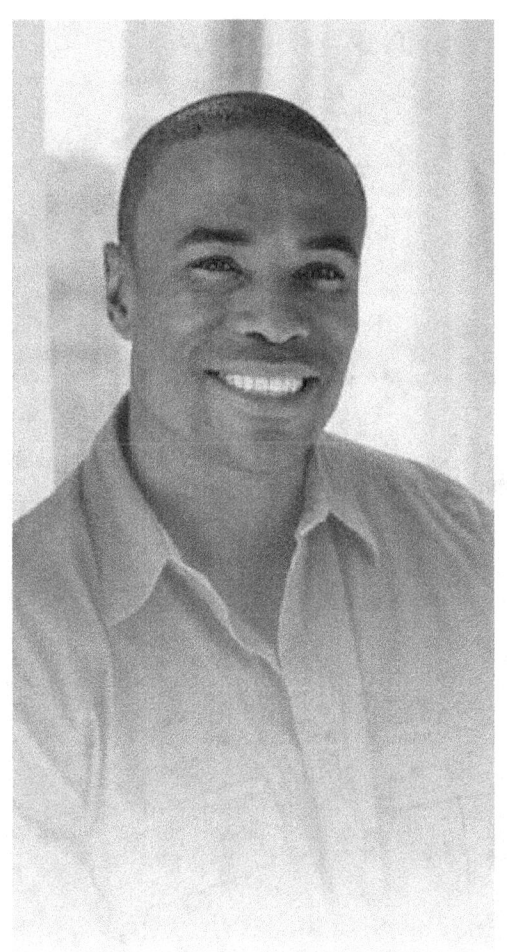

In response to these opportunities, DHAP staff undertook the development of a strategic plan focused on Division activities (see sidebar to learn more about the development process). Applying lessons learned from previous CDC-wide plans, and recommendations from an April 2009 External Peer Review that laid the foundation for a Division-specific plan, DHAP sought to create a framework for operations, concentrating on the Division's role in preventing HIV. The result of this process, DHAP's Strategic Plan 2011-2015 (the Plan), provides an unprecedented opportunity for the Division to achieve high-impact prevention by strengthening both its internal operations and its work with governmental and non-governmental partners to advance national and organizational goals and objectives.

Targeting Hard-Hit Communities: The Enhanced Comprehensive HIV Prevention Planning Project

A significant component of the plan developed by the U.S. Department of Health and Human Services (HHS) to operationalize the National HIV/AIDS Strategy is its "Twelve Cities Project," an effort to support comprehensive planning and cross agency response in 12 communities hit hard by AIDS. The initiative actively engages multiple agencies within HHS and is anchored by DHAP's Enhanced Comprehensive HIV Prevention Planning (ECHPP) project. ECHPP launched in September 2010, when DHAP awarded grants totaling $11.6 million to support demonstration projects to identify and implement a "combination approach" to enhance effective HIV prevention programming in targeted communities. These efforts both supplemented existing programs and helped better focus efforts on key at-risk populations.

The funded jurisdictions—New York City, Los Angeles, District of Columbia, Chicago, Georgia, Florida, Philadelphia, Houston, San Francisco, Maryland, Texas, and Puerto Rico—are working with DHAP staff to determine what mix of HIV prevention approaches can have the greatest impact in the local area based on the local profile of the epidemic and assessment of current gaps in their HIV prevention portfolios. While the exact combination of approaches will vary by area, efforts funded under this program will follow a basic approach of: expanding HIV testing to reduce undiagnosed HIV infection; prioritizing linkage, retention, and quality of care and prevention services for people living with HIV; and directing these intensified efforts to communities with the highest burden of HIV.

ECHPP represents a game-changing effort by DHAP to support a more coordinated response to HIV at the local level and demonstrates DHAP's commitment to maximizing the impact and efficiency of HIV prevention efforts and implementing the NHAS mandate to target prevention to communities and geographic areas where HIV is most heavily concentrated. ECHPP expands efforts to reduce HIV incidence, improve the health of people living with HIV, and reduce HIV-related disparities by using a combination of cost-effective, evidence-based approaches that can be scaled to meet local needs.

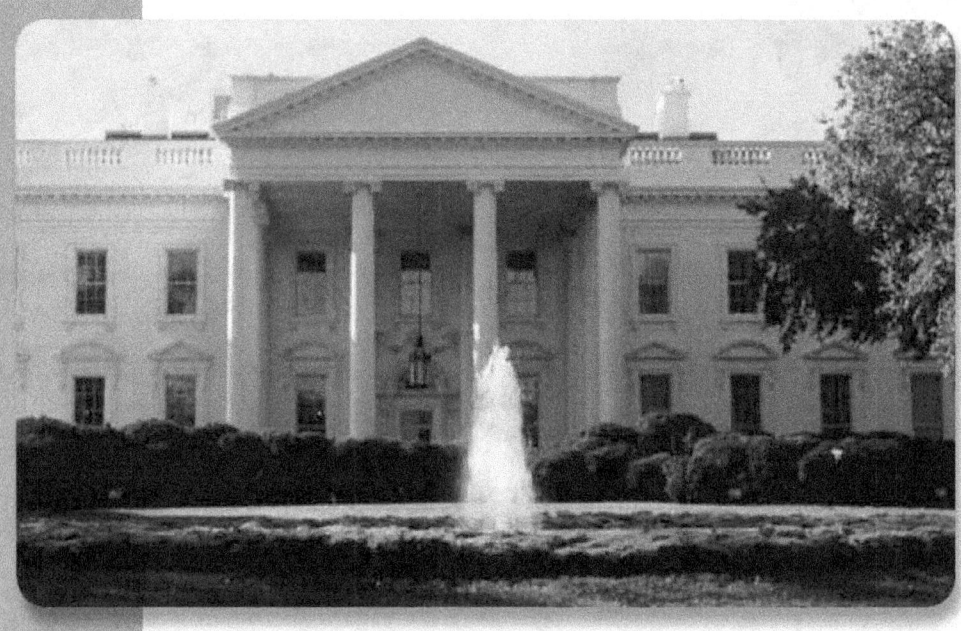

Echoing the Priorities of the National HIV/AIDS Strategy and the NCHHSTP Strategic Plan 2010-2015

DHAP's Plan was influenced by the Division's participation in the White House Office of National AIDS Policy's process for developing the National HIV/AIDS Strategy (NHAS). Working through NCHHSTP and the Office of the Secretary in the U.S. Department of Health and Human Services (HHS), DHAP staff served on key committees responsible for drafting NHAS. The input of these same staff during the development of the Plan ensured it was aligned with NHAS and set a course for the Division that furthered the goals and objectives of the broader strategy.

The Plan also echoes the priorities articulated in the NCHHSTP Strategic Plan 2010-2015 released in March 2010. For example, the Plan supports increased linkage to and retention in care as a prevention strategy and emphasizes the need to coordinate and support appropriate collaboration between HIV prevention programs and efforts addressing other co-morbid conditions, including other sexually transmitted diseases (STDs), viral hepatitis, and tuberculosis. For additional information on the links among the Plan, NHAS and the NCHHSTP Strategic Plan, see Appendix C.

The Process for Developing the DHAP Strategic Plan 2011-2015

The foundation for DHAP's Plan was established at a meeting held in April 2009, when the Division, under the auspices of CDC's Board of Scientific Counselors, convened an External Peer Review of DHAP Surveillance, Research and HIV Prevention.[1] This intensive examination of DHAP activities created an opportunity to obtain input and guidance on the Division's scientific and programmatic priorities and strategic direction in order to draft a strategic plan focused solely on DHAP.

Participants in the External Peer Review—including academicians, health professionals, state health department staff, representatives from affected communities, and representatives from nongovernmental organizations—were divided into five panels:

1. Planning, Prioritizing, and Monitoring
2. Surveillance
3. Biomedical Interventions, Diagnostics, Laboratory, and Health Services Research
4. Behavioral, Social, and Structural Interventions Research
5. Prevention Programs, Capacity Building, and Program Evaluation.

Each panel examined the following aspects of DHAP programs that fell within its purview: relevance to DHAP mission; scope and relative priority; scientific and technical quality, approach, and direction; adequacy of translation and dissemination of research findings for use in programs; strengths, gaps, challenges, and opportunities; and extent to which the activity addresses the NCHHSTP imperatives of program collaboration and service integration and reducing health disparities. In November 2009, DHAP published a response to the final recommendations made by the participants at the end of the External Peer Review (available online at www.cdc.gov/hiv/strategic_planning/exec_summary.htm).

Building on the success of the External Peer Review, in early 2010, 80 senior DHAP leaders (e.g., the Division Director, Deputy Directors, Associate Directors, branch chiefs, team leads, and other senior staff) participated in a 2½ day retreat to define the Division's vision and mission and to identify the goals and objectives of the Plan. These leaders twice reconvened for additional 2-day planning meetings, refining objectives and strategies. During the summer and fall of 2010, staff representing a broad cross section of the Division continued to review drafts and provide feedback. DHAP formed several work groups to focus on finalizing specific aspects of the Plan. DHAP also conducted two Division-wide employee surveys, the first in February/March 2010 and a second in November 2010.

Honoring its promise to undertake a transparent strategic planning process, DHAP consulted external stakeholders throughout the development process. Early in the process, DHAP conducted face-to-face and telephone interviews with 49 key internal and external leaders. As worked progress, the Division continued to seek input, using as a sounding board a Strategic Plan External Work Group comprised of the DHAP external partners who had served on the External Peer Review Steering Committee. At each stage in this process, comments were carefully considered and incorporated into a subsequent draft.

From these sessions emerged a Plan with a new vision and mission for the Division. This new vision—a future free of HIV—describes in words the world DHAP hopes to move toward in implementing the Plan. This will come about by DHAP fulfilling its mission: promoting health and quality of life by preventing HIV infection and reducing HIV-related illness and death in the United States.

[1] The external review was implemented by CDC to ensure agency compliance with Office of Management and Budget "Guidelines for Ensuring and Maximizing the Quality, Objectivity, Utility, and Integrity of Information Disseminated by Federal Agencies."

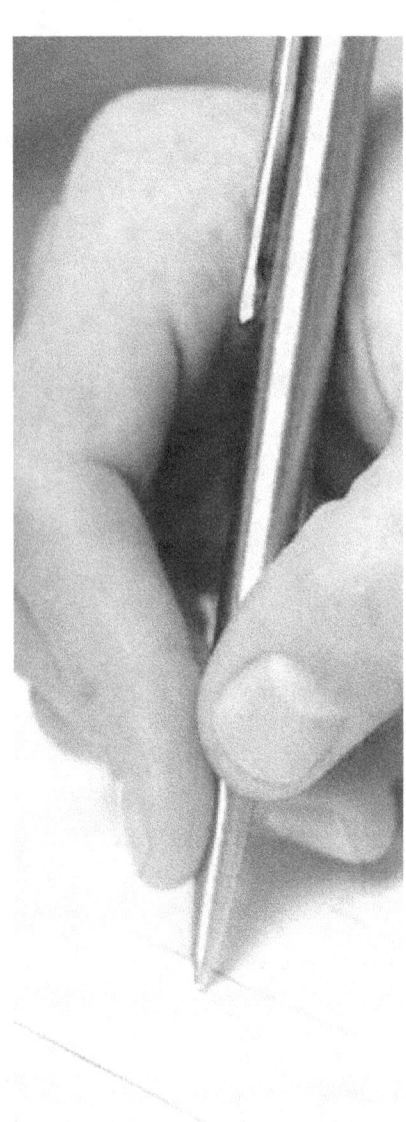

The Plan

DHAP's Strategic Plan 2011-2015 consists of 4 goals, 20 objectives, and 14 strategies focused specifically on strengthening DHAP programming and operations (see Appendix B for an easy-to-read reference chart of the goals, objectives, and strategies). Each goal is a broadly-stated idea that captures the core of what DHAP plans to accomplish: reduce HIV incidence, link individuals who test positive into care so that they can remain healthy and prevent transmission, reduce disparities, and achieve organizational excellence. For each goal, objectives provide specific and quantifiable measures that will allow DHAP to gauge its progress toward meeting the goals outlined in the Plan. Finally, strategies are broadly-stated activities required to achieve the goals and objectives.

Achieving High-Impact Prevention

Based on feedback from DHAP staff and internal and external stakeholders as to how the strategic planning process could best serve the Division, the Plan encompasses all activity within the Division and focuses on strengthening internal operations. This comprehensive structure best aligns with DHAP's desire to ensure all of its work is mapped to specific organizational goals, objectives, and strategies.

In the Plan, key functions of the Division—such as surveillance, research, and programs—remain the same. What is new is the systematic and deliberative approach the Division will take to accomplish and coordinate these activities. Within each area as well as across functions, the Plan focuses on prioritizing activities based on their effectiveness, cost, coverage, feasibility, and scalability. This ensures DHAP is best allocating its limited resources to achieve high-impact prevention.

Top priorities for implementation are:

- Making prioritized recommendations for maintaining critical surveillance systems, filling knowledge gaps, increasing capacity, and reducing redundancies
- Better identifying current drivers of HIV incidence and using this research to design and target interventions and strategies
- Developing and implementing a framework for more effectively integrating and using data to evaluate HIV prevention activities and their impact and to guide the national response
- Creating a unified research agenda that encompasses prevention of new infections and increasing linkage to and impact of prevention and care services for people living with HIV
- Improving mathematical models and economic analyses to explore the best combination of prevention activities
- Developing comprehensive internal and external communication plans and creating an external partnership framework and inventory to guide partner engagement
- Strengthening allocation and management processes for extramural resources to improve accountability and maximize DHAP's impact on the HIV epidemic.

The Plan recognizes that all effective interventions are not equal and that, given resource limitations, DHAP must prioritize its work, applying the science of implementation to maximize impact.

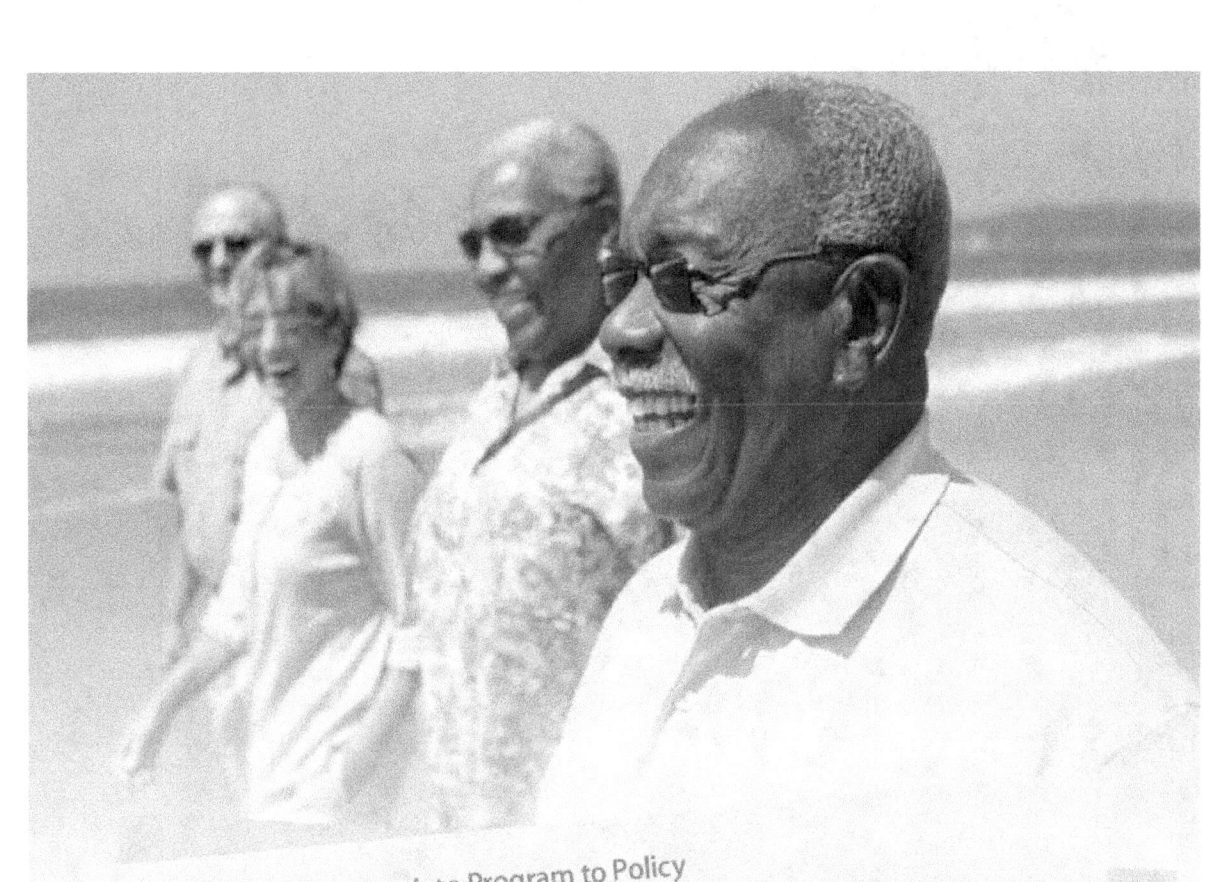

Moving from Research to Program to Policy

New approaches are urgently needed to prevent HIV infections. This means that promising strategies must move from research to program to policy in record time. DHAP is well-positioned to contribute to this continuum, illustrated by its participation in conducting research and supporting clinical trials to evaluate the safety and efficacy of pre-exposure prophylaxis (PrEP).

In late 2010, findings from one of these trials were released, indicating that PrEP, when combined with other comprehensive prevention approaches, was safe and effective in preventing HIV among men who have sex with men (MSM) who are at high risk of infection. DHAP responded to these findings by pursuing two primary goals: developing guidance on the safe and effective use of PrEP among MSM, and determining how to most effectively use PrEP in combination with other prevention strategies to reduce new infections among MSM in the United States.

In late January 2011, CDC released interim guidance for physicians on prescribing PrEP to prevent HIV among high-risk MSM. CDC is also serving as the lead federal agency in developing U.S. Public Health Service PrEP guidelines, in collaboration with other federal health agencies. The guidelines will be based on a full review of trial data and other research, and will incorporate input from health care providers, HIV prevention partners, and affected communities. The guidelines will help ensure both physicians and MSM have accurate information to guide decisions about the use of PrEP.

Recognizing opportunities to expand the portfolio of prevention tools and acting quickly to move these opportunities from research to program to policy is essential to achieving high-impact prevention and an integral component of DHAP's Strategic Plan 2011-2015.

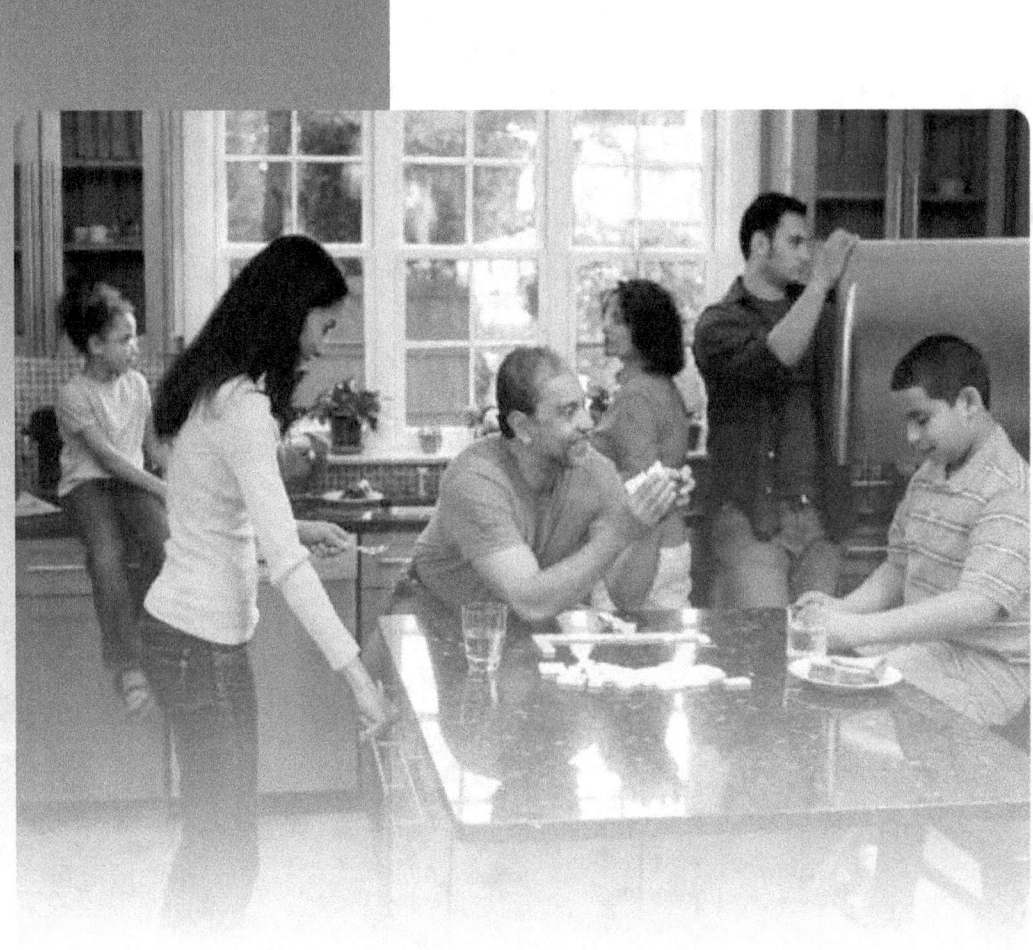

The Plan Goals and Objectives

GOAL A: HIV Incidence—Prevent new infections

Goal A and its corresponding objectives and strategies are focused primarily on prevention with people who have not been diagnosed with HIV but who are at high risk for infection, and identifying persons previously unaware of their HIV infection. The four strategies in Goal A encompass many of DHAP's traditional roles related to surveillance and program research and implementation. They are:

- A1: Systematically collect, analyze, integrate, and disseminate data to monitor the HIV epidemic, assess the impact of HIV prevention activities, and guide the national response;

- A2: Identify drivers of HIV incidence in priority populations (as identified in NHAS) to design and target effective interventions and strategies for maximum impact;

- A3: Identify, develop and evaluate effective behavioral, biomedical and structural technologies, interventions and strategies; prioritize this process to maximize reduction of HIV acquisition among high-incidence populations;

- A4: Implement and evaluate effective behavioral, structural, and biomedical technologies, interventions and strategies at scale; prioritize and target implementation to maximally reduce HIV acquisition in high-incidence populations.

GOAL A: HIV INCIDENCE—Prevent New Infections

Objective 1*
By 2015, reduce the annual number of new HIV infections by 25%

Objective 2*
By 2015, increase the percentage of people living with HIV who know their serostatus to 90%

Objective 3
By 2015, increase the percentage of people diagnosed with HIV infection at earlier stages of disease (not stage 3: AIDS), by 25%

Objective 4
By 2015, decrease the rate of perinatally acquired pediatric HIV cases by 25%

Objective 5
By 2015, reduce the proportion of MSM who reported unprotected anal intercourse during their last sexual encounter with a partner of discordant or unknown HIV status by 25%

Objective 6
By 2015, reduce the proportion of IDU who reported risky sexual or drug using behavior by 25%

Strategy A1
Systematically collect, analyze, integrate, and disseminate data to monitor the HIV epidemic, assess the impact of HIV prevention activities, and guide the national response

Strategy A2
Identify drivers of HIV incidence in priority populations (as identified in NHAS) to design and target effective interventions and strategies for maximum impact

Strategy A3
Identify, develop and evaluate effective behavioral, biomedical and structural technologies, interventions and strategies; prioritize this process to maximize reduction of HIV acquisition among high-incidence populations

Strategy A4
Implement and evaluate effective behavioral, structural, and biomedical technologies, interventions and strategies at scale; prioritize and target implementation to maximally reduce HIV acquisition in high-incidence populations

*Objective taken from NHAS

The first strategy, A1, focuses on DHAP's surveillance activities and builds on the Division's expertise in this area. Tasks DHAP will undertake to strengthen its surveillance program include developing and applying a framework for integrating and using data to guide the national response and evaluating the impact of HIV prevention activities. DHAP will also work to increase the capacity for effective and timely use of DHAP data by national, state, and local partners.

Strategy A2 calls on DHAP to further investigate possible drivers of the domestic HIV epidemic—such as social and economic determinants of health (e.g., racism, poverty, stigma, and low education) and access to care and prevention services—and integrate what is learned into DHAP surveillance, research, and program activities.

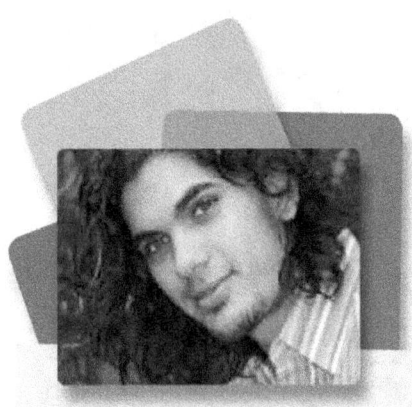

Community Viral Load Surveillance: A new tool for targeting prevention

Community viral load (CVL), defined as the mean or total viral load (amount of the virus in the blood) of all HIV positive individuals receiving care in a given area, has been associated with HIV incidence. Monitoring CVL, while mapping and modeling other aspects of HIV, creates new opportunities to respond to local epidemics. For example, in areas where CVL is high and likelihood of transmission greater, programs and services can be targeted to ensure people living with HIV are linked to and maintained in care and adhere to appropriate and timely medical and prevention services to decrease their viral load.

To assist jurisdictions in implementing this targeted approach, DHAP provides national leadership, financial resources, and technical assistance. Health jurisdictions funded by DHAP for surveillance receive support to collect viral load data and develop local CVL estimates as well as calculate the proportion of people with HIV linked to and retained in care. DHAP also provides support to improve the ability of health departments to use geospatial information to monitor and respond to the local epidemic.

Viral load and CD4 cell count data are also helpful in monitoring the effectiveness of HIV prevention programs. In 2010, DHAP began funding 3 year demonstration projects in the District of Columbia and the Bronx in New York City to develop, monitor, and evaluate models for using CVL and other surveillance data to improve the effectiveness of local HIV prevention.

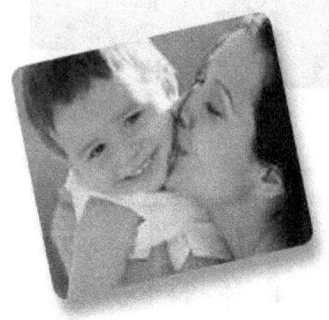

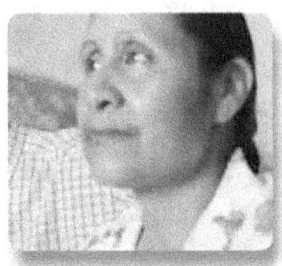

The final two strategies focus on identifying, implementing, and evaluating effective behavioral, biomedical and structural technologies and interventions to prevent new HIV infections. Key activities planned as part of these strategies are:

- Create a Division-wide, prioritized research agenda;
- Develop mathematical models and conduct economic analyses to explore the best combinations of prevention activities, interventions, and strategies;
- Create a mechanism that would ensure research findings inform program development and implementation and that programmatic needs inform research directions;
- Prioritize prevention activities and implement based on that prioritization;
- Monitor and evaluate implementation of prevention activities to improve program performance

Reducing Incidence: Prevention with People Living with HIV

Prevention with people living with HIV (PWP) is a key component of the DHAP Strategic Plan 2011-2015 in recognition that reducing transmission is critical to meeting its 2015 targets. Current activities include working with the Health Resources and Services Administration (HRSA) and others on updating CDC's 2003 PWP recommendations. The revised recommendations focus on a comprehensive approach: linkage to and retention in care; risk assessment and drug use and sexual risk reduction services; treatment as prevention; adherence to treatment; and other aspects. The recommendations will also include prevention in both health care and non-health care settings.

Co-sponsors for the revision include governmental and non-governmental partners such as the National Institutes of Health (NIH), the HIV Medical Association, the American Academy of HIV Medicine, the National Association of People with AIDS, and the National Minority AIDS Council.

PWP is also a focus of other DHAP activities. For example, the Enhanced Comprehensive HIV Prevention Planning project (ECHPP) requires grantees to prioritize prevention and linkage to care for people living with HIV. In line with integrating prevention and care services, DHAP's Prevention Research Synthesis project recently published a list of evidence-based HIV medication adherence interventions.

GOAL B: Prevention and Care—Increase linkage to and impact of prevention and care services with people living with HIV/AIDS

Goal B and its corresponding objectives and strategies are focused primarily on prevention with people who have been diagnosed with HIV. It emphasizes DHAP working with and through the health care delivery system to implement interventions to decrease transmission risk and increase retention in care and adherence to treatment regimens. Goal B strategies are:

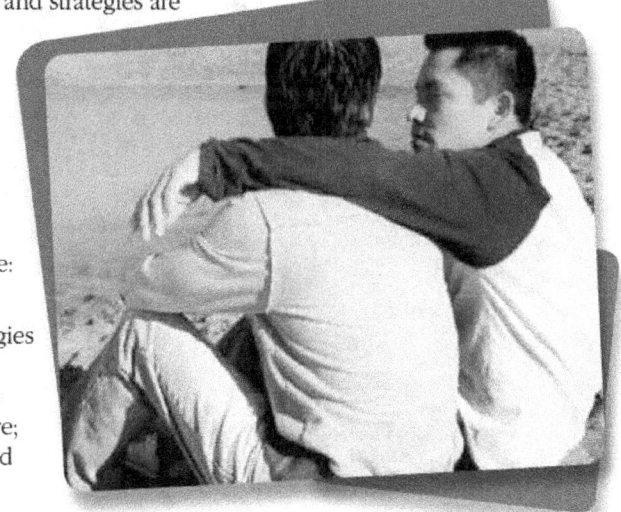

- B1: Identify, develop, and evaluate interventions, strategies, and technologies to increase linkage to care and use of antiretroviral therapy (ART); maximize adherence to ART and retention in care; reduce transmission risk behaviors; and provide partner services;

- B2: Ensure the implementation and evaluation of interventions, strategies, and technologies to increase linkage to care and use of ART; maximize adherence to ART and retention in care; reduce transmission risk behaviors; and provide partner services.

GOAL B: PREVENTION AND CARE—Increase Linkage to and Impact of Prevention and Care Services with People Living with HIV/AIDS

Objective 1*
By 2015, reduce the HIV transmission rate by 30%

Objective 2*
By 2015, increase the percentage of persons diagnosed with HIV who are linked to clinical care as evidenced by having a CD4 count or viral load measure within 3 months of HIV diagnosis to 85%

Objective 3
By 2015, increase by 10% the percentage of HIV-diagnosed persons in care whose most recent viral load test in the past 12 months was undetectable

Objective 4
By 2015, reduce the percentage of HIV-diagnosed persons in care who report unprotected anal or vaginal intercourse during the last 12 months with partners of discordant or unknown HIV status by 33%

Strategy B1
Identify, develop, and evaluate interventions, strategies, and technologies to increase linkage to care and use of ART; maximize adherence to ART and retention in care; reduce transmission risk behaviors; and provide partner services

Strategy B2
Ensure the implementation and evaluation of interventions, strategies, and technologies to increase linkage to care and use of ART; maximize adherence to ART and retention in care; reduce transmission risk behaviors; and provide partner services

*Objective taken from NHAS

Many Goal B activities both relate to and interact with those activities implemented under Goal A. For example, research prioritized under strategy B1 will link to activities under Goal A related to creating a unified research agenda. In addition, the implementation and evaluation of interventions, strategies, and technologies in strategy B2 includes monitoring coverage and outcomes that will link to Goal A surveillance activities. Despite this anticipated interaction between Goal A and Goal B, separating the two allowed the Division to craft objectives and strategies targeted specifically to prevention with people living with HIV. This acknowledges the critical role of public health in linking individuals to treatment and ensuring prevention services are integrated in care for people living with HIV/AIDS.

GOAL C: Health Disparities—Reduce HIV-related disparities

Goal C and its corresponding objectives and strategies are focused primarily on ensuring the reduction of HIV-related disparities as well as developing partnerships and ensuring DHAP activities are culturally and linguistically appropriate. Goal C strategies are:

- C1: Target resources and activities to reduce HIV-related disparities (through Goals A and B);
- C2: Monitor national trends and DHAP activities and outcomes to ensure that HIV-related disparities and their underlying factors are reduced (through Goals A and B);
- C3: Communicate DHAP activities and progress to stakeholders and enlist partners to advance activities that reduce disparities (to be coordinated with Strategy D2 partnership engagement framework);
- C4: Ensure the cultural and linguistic appropriateness of DHAP activities and materials to increase their impact.

Pursuing Health Equity

HIV does not affect all populations equally—95% of people living with AIDS in the United States are men who have sex with men, African Americans, Latinos, or injection drug users. Responding to these tremendous disparities, in September 2010, DHAP established an Office of Health Equity (OHE) to coordinate and monitor the Division's activities related to reducing health inequities among populations and risk groups disproportionately affected by HIV.

OHE priorities include:

- Providing leadership to the Division's efforts to document HIV and AIDS inequities, understand their determinants, and craft strategies for increasing health equity.
- Collaborating with the NCHHSTP Office of Health Equity and other CDC components focused on addressing health inequities.
- Serving as the Division liaison with key stakeholder groups including, but not limited to, state and local public health officials, community-based organizations, policy makers, and advocates on HIV and AIDS issues related to health inequities.
- Developing partnerships with other federal and non-governmental organizations focused on addressing HIV and AIDS issues related to health inequities.

OHE will play a large role in implementing the DHAP Strategic Plan 2011 2015, monitoring the Division's performance on objectives related to HIV inequities and working with staff to integrate methods for addressing health inequities into program activities.

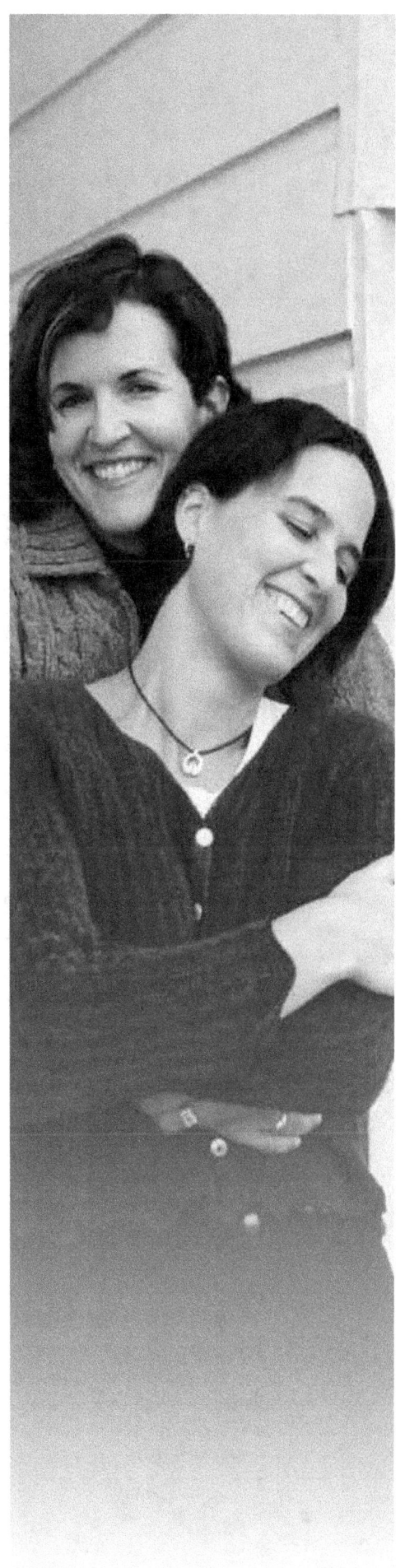

GOAL C: HEALTH DISPARITIES—Reduce HIV-Related Disparities

Objective 1*
By 2015, increase the percentage of HIV-diagnosed MSM with undetectable viral load by 20%

Objective 2*
By 2015, increase the percentage of HIV-diagnosed Blacks with undetectable viral load by 20%

Objective 3*
By 2015, increase the percentage of HIV-diagnosed Hispanics with undetectable viral load by 20%

Objective 4
By 2015, reduce the annual number of new HIV infections among MSM, Blacks, Hispanics and IDU by at least 25% in each group

Objective 5
By 2015, ensure the percentage of persons diagnosed with HIV who have a CD4 count within 3 months of HIV diagnosis is 75% or greater for all racial/ethnic groups

Strategy C1
Target resources and activities to reduce HIV-related disparities (through Goals A and B)

Strategy C2
Monitor national trends and DHAP activities and outcomes to ensure that HIV-related disparities and their underlying factors are reduced (through Goals A and B)

Strategy C3
Communicate DHAP activities and progress to stakeholders and enlist partners to advance activities that reduce disparities (to be coordinated with Strategy D2 partnership engagement framework)

Strategy C4
Ensure the cultural and linguistic appropriateness of DHAP activities and materials to increase their impact

*Objective taken from NHAS

The first two strategies empower DHAP staff charged with implementing Goal C to interact and partner with leaders for the other strategies to ensure DHAP surveillance, research, and program activities are appropriately targeted. This will occur through the development of standards to assess the degree to which research agendas and program activities carried out under the Plan are both informed by and adequately address and prioritize disproportionately affected populations and risk groups.

The third strategy calls for partnership and communications activities focused specifically on reducing HIV-related disparities. This strategy directs DHAP staff to develop a plan for communicating information about the Division's progress toward achieving its disparities-related objectives and to reach out to key partners and stakeholders to gather input into DHAP activities and to disseminate HIV-prevention messages to affected communities.

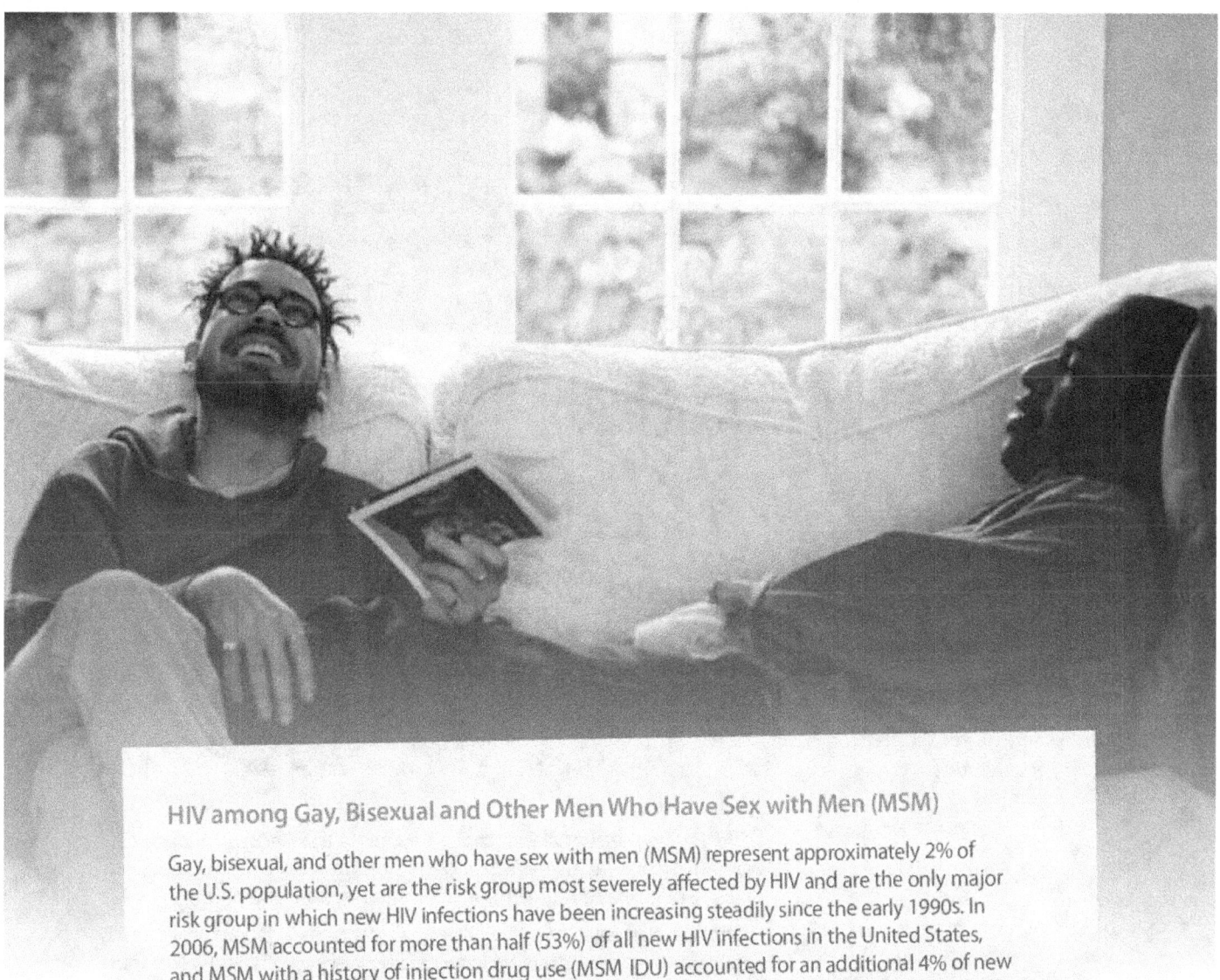

HIV among Gay, Bisexual and Other Men Who Have Sex with Men (MSM)

Gay, bisexual, and other men who have sex with men (MSM) represent approximately 2% of the U.S. population, yet are the risk group most severely affected by HIV and are the only major risk group in which new HIV infections have been increasing steadily since the early 1990s. In 2006, MSM accounted for more than half (53%) of all new HIV infections in the United States, and MSM with a history of injection drug use (MSM IDU) accounted for an additional 4% of new infections.[1] The high prevalence of HIV infection among MSM means they face a greater risk of being exposed to infection with each sexual encounter, especially as they get older.

To decrease this risk, DHAP targets a significant portion of its funding—43% in fiscal year 2009—to preventing HIV among MSM, a proportion DHAP intends to increase. DHAP also conducts research to better understand the factors that lead to HIV infection and identify effective approaches to prevent infection among MSM, including expanded HIV testing and linkage to care. Finally, CDC partners with national, regional and community organizations and media outlets serving the gay community to increase awareness of HIV and to improve the sexual health of MSM.

For more information, please go to: http://www.cdc.gov/hiv/topics/msm.

[1] Hall HI, Song R, Rhodes P, et al. Estimation of HIV incidence in the United States. JAMA 2008;300(5):520 529.

Finally, strategy C4 instructs DHAP to ensure cultural and linguistic appropriateness of its activities. This includes assessing research proposals, educational materials, and program activities, revising or developing new materials as necessary, and providing resources to Division staff to increase their cultural sensitivity and cultural competency.

Educating the Nation about HIV

Launched in 2009, Act Against AIDS (AAA) is a 5-year, national communication campaign to refocus attention on the domestic HIV/AIDS epidemic and mobilize leaders to take steps to prevent AIDS in their own communities, with an emphasis on populations and risk groups bearing a disproportionate burden of HIV/AIDS, such as African American, Hispanic and Latino communities and men of all races and ethnicities who have sex with other men (MSM). Each phase will be focused on different audiences and use mass media and direct-to-consumer communication efforts to deliver prevention messages that are compelling, credible, and relevant.

One example is the *Know Where You Stand* campaign, which is focused on increasing testing among Black men who have sex with men, one of the populations most affected by HIV. Another campaign, *Prevention is Care*, targets providers who deliver care to patients living with HIV, encouraging them to screen their patients for transmission risk behaviors and to deliver brief prevention messages on the importance of reducing such behaviors. Finally, the *I Know* campaign seeks to raise awareness about the importance of talking about HIV testing, condom use, and myths and misperceptions about HIV with peers, partners, and families of African American men and women aged 18 to 24.

Learn more about AAA at: www.cdc.gov/hiv/aaa.

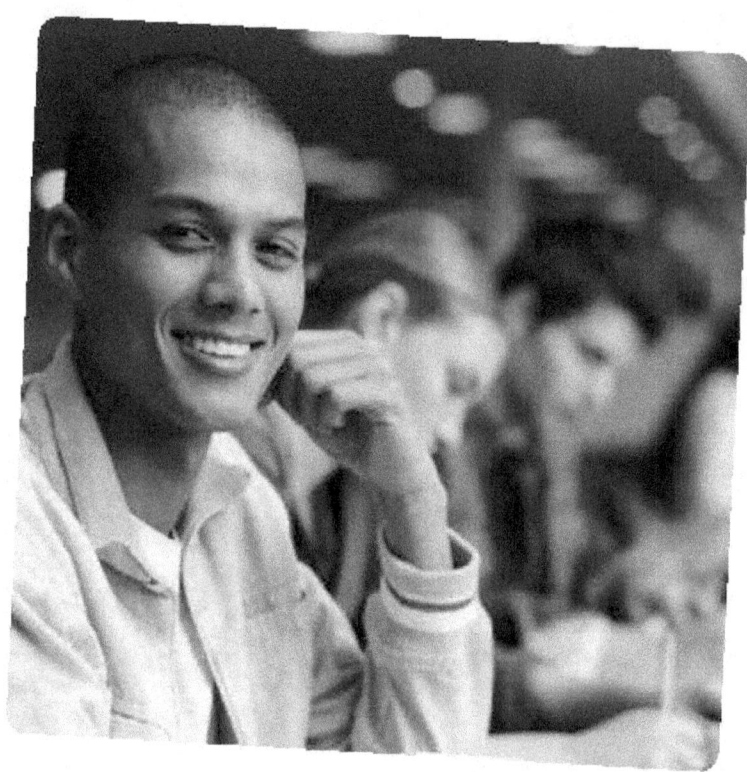

GOAL D: Organizational Excellence—Promote a skilled and engaged workforce and effective, efficient operations to ensure the successful delivery of CDC's HIV prevention science, programs and policies

Optimal implementation of the other goals demands organizational excellence, key elements of which support all aspects of DHAP programs. Through Goal D, DHAP will pursue the following strategies:

* D1: Develop, implement and monitor an internal communication plan with two-way communication channels to improve transparency, accountability, participation and coordination both within DHAP and with other CDC stakeholders;

* D2: Develop, implement and monitor an external communication and partner engagement plan to improve transparency, accountability, participation and collaboration through bi-directional flow of information;

* D3: Maximize the effectiveness of DHAP human and financial resources to achieve DHAP's strategic goals and objectives;

* D4: Allocate extramural resources and use results-oriented management to improve accountability and maximize the impact of all DHAP-supported activities on the HIV epidemic.

GOAL D: ORGANIZATIONAL EXCELLENCE—
Promote a Skilled and Engaged Workforce and Effective,
Efficient Operations to Ensure the Successful Delivery
of CDC's HIV Prevention Science, Programs and Policies

Objective 1
Each year, all branches and operating units will complete at least 80% of their work plan activities

Objective 2
Each year, all branches and operating units will adhere to 80% of their administrative and extramural processing deadlines

Objective
By 2015, DHAP will have improved its rating on the HHS Annual Employee Viewpoint Survey

Strategy D1
Develop, implement and monitor an internal communication plan with two-way communication channels to improve transparency, accountability, participation and coordination both within DHAP and with other CDC stakeholders

Strategy D2
Develop, implement and monitor an external communication and partner engagement plan to improve transparency, accountability, participation and collaboration through bi-directional flow of information

Strategy D3
Maximize the effectiveness of DHAP human and financial resources to achieve DHAP's strategic goals and objectives

Strategy D4
Allocate extramural resources and use results-oriented management to improve accountability and maximize the impact of all DHAP-supported activities on the HIV epidemic

The first two strategies focus on DHAP's internal and external communication activities, tasking the Division with being transparent, accountable and collaborative. Emphasis is placed not just on diffusing messages but creating feedback loops to learn from partners.

Partnering to Reach Communities at Greatest Risk

Coordination and collaboration with external partners are highlighted as essential to successful implementation throughout DHAP's Strategic Plan 2011 2015. An example of DHAP's commitment to partnership is the Act Against AIDS Leadership Initiative (AAALI), launched as part of the Act Against AIDS communication campaign. AAALI is a 6 year partnership with leading national organizations representing populations hardest hit by HIV. Chosen for their demonstrated national reach, credibility, and influence, AAALI brings together a wide range of organizations, including civic, social, civil rights and professional organizations, as well as those in government, education and media.

Since April 2009, AAALI partner organizations have coordinated more than 1,400 outreach events attended by more than 200,000 people; engaged nearly 400 local affiliates across the country in HIV prevention activities; and reached millions more with critical HIV prevention messages through conferences, advertisements and media stories. In addition, AAALI has generated approximately 170 million media impressions.

Learn more about AAALI at:
www.cdc.gov/hiv/aaa/leadership initiative.htm.

Under Strategy D3, DHAP will monitor and evaluate its activities to ensure alignment with Division priorities. Branches and operating units will develop detailed work plans that will map projects to specific Division goals and objectives. These work plans will allow DHAP to closely track internal performance and guide allocation of resources across the Plan's activities. Strategy D3 also emphasizes developing and implementing plans for recruiting and retaining highly qualified staff and ensuring continuous growth and learning opportunities to help staff better perform their jobs.

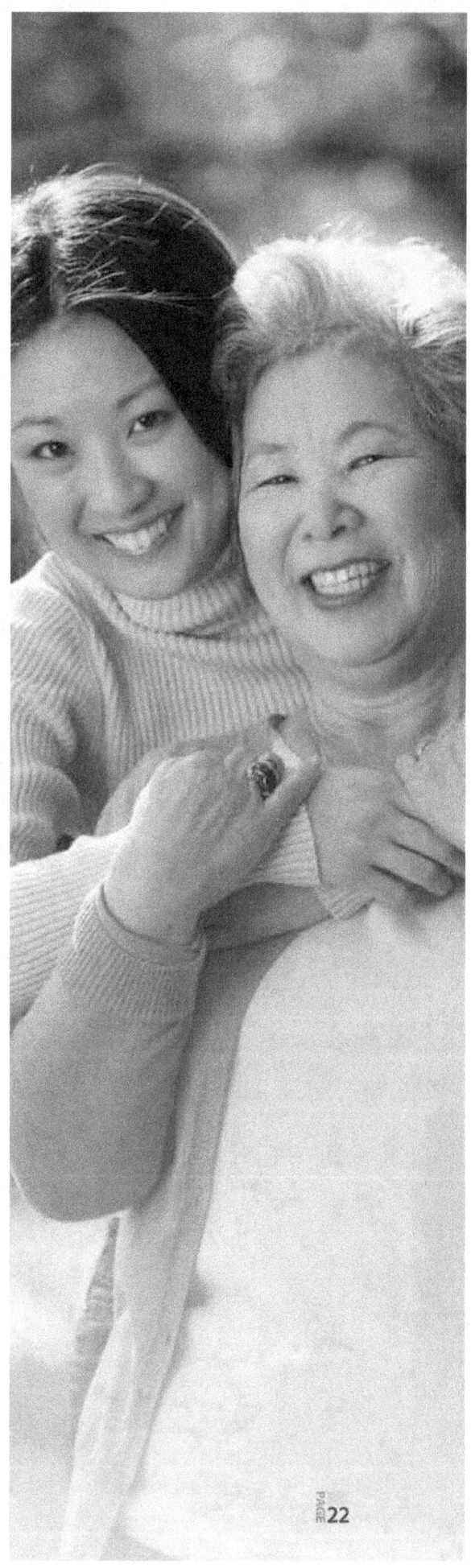

Allocating Funding to Achieve High-Impact Prevention

The U.S. HIV epidemic continues to be concentrated in specific geographic areas, with marked racial, ethnic, social, and economic disparities. While HIV prevention activities have achieved some success among certain populations, incidence among men who have sex with men (MSM) is increasing. In response, DHAP is adopting new approaches to allocate its limited prevention funding.

For example, beginning in 2012, the Division will use a new algorithm to allocate funding to state and local health departments. This program—representing approximately half of DHAP's entire budget—provides the foundation for HIV prevention and control nationwide. Funding will support:

- Delivering of effective, evidence-based biomedical and behavioral prevention interventions to reduce HIV incidence, including promoting HIV testing and linkage to care, and re-engagement into care of previously diagnosed HIV-positive individuals
- Implementing interventions with individuals who are HIV-positive including use of and adherence to antiretroviral therapy, partner services, and behavioral risk reduction
- Targeting services to populations at highest risk for HIV acquisition with scalable, culturally appropriate interventions.

Under the new funding algorithm, core funding will be provided to all health department jurisdictions to allow basic program activities to continue (e.g., testing of persons at high risk, linkage to care, partner services) but funding above core will be distributed based on need. The main criterion used for the algorithm will be the number of people diagnosed and reported to be living with HIV infection during 2008, the latest year for which data are available.

Health departments that distribute CDC funding will also adjust how they allocate funds, placing greater emphasis on effective interventions for people living with HIV as well as effective community-level, structural and single-session interventions and public health strategies. Intensive individual and small group interventions for at-risk populations that are difficult to take to scale will be de-emphasized. Funding realignments will be phased in over 5 years to minimize disruption to grantee activities and allow for planning. Use of the new algorithm and redirection of funding from less effective and efficient interventions to interventions that are aligned with the goals of the DHAP Strategic Plan 2011-2015 and NHAS will help achieve high-impact prevention.

Learn more about DHAP funding opportunities at: www.cdc.gov/hiv/topics/funding

The final strategy under Goal D addresses how DHAP operates in relation to its external partners. To achieve high-impact prevention, it is critical that DHAP maximize its extramural resources, allocating funds based on an HIV epidemic that is increasingly concentrated in specific geographic areas and marked by racial, ethnic, social, and economic disparities. The Division must also establish and enforce expectations for performance among its grantees, providing guidance and support to build local capacity and using standardized review criteria to evaluate effectiveness.

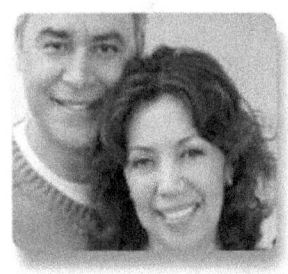

Next Steps

Over the next months, senior leaders in the Division will work with DHAP staff to implement the Plan with a 6-month target that all activities occuring in the Division will be mapped to a specific goal, objective and strategy.

DHAP is committed to achieving high-impact prevention—to prioritizing the allocation of prevention resources, careful monitoring and constant re-evaluation, targeted research, and intensive and sustained collaboration and coordination with partners. The Plan is the framework that will make this possible, enabling the Division to focus on its specific role in preventing HIV and accelerating progress toward accomplishing its goals and objectives.

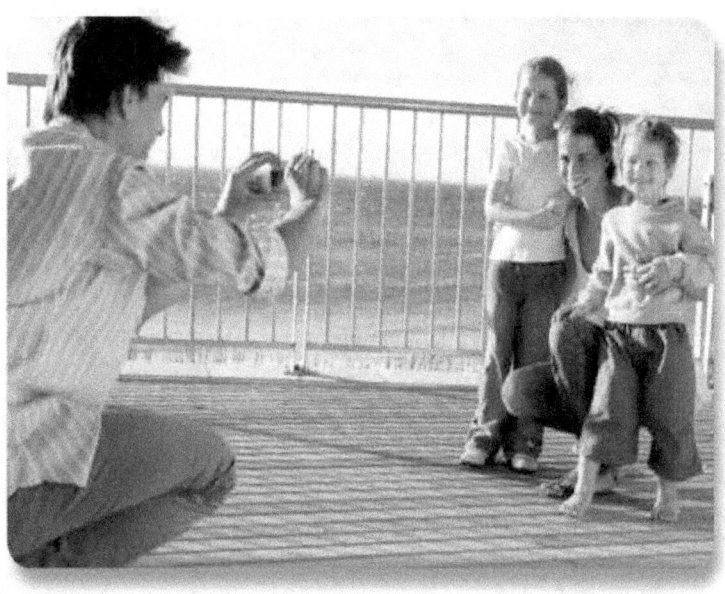

Appendix A — List of Acronyms

AAA: Act Against AIDS

AAALI: Act Against AIDS Leadership Initiative

AIDS: Acquired Immunodeficiency Syndrome

ART: Anti-retroviral therapy

CDC: Centers for Disease Control and Prevention

CVL: Community viral load

DHAP: Division of HIV/AIDS Prevention

EBI: Effective behavioral interventions

ECHPP: Enhanced Comprehensive HIV Prevention Planning project

HHS: U.S. Department of Health and Human Services

HIV: Human Immunodeficiency Virus

HRSA: Health Resources and Services Administration

IHS: Indian Health Service

IDU: Injection drug users

MSM: Men who have sex with men

MSM-IDU: Men with a history of injection drug use who have sex with men

NHAS: National HIV/AIDS Strategy

NIH: National Institutes of Health

NCHHSTP: National Center for HIV/AIDS, Viral Hepatitis, STD, and TB Prevention

OHE: Office of Health Equity in DHAP

PrEP: Pre-exposure prophylaxis

PWP: Prevention with people living with HIV

STDs: Sexually transmitted diseases

Appendix B — Goal, Objectives, and Strategies

GOAL A: HIV INCIDENCE—Prevent New Infections

Objective 1*
By 2015, reduce the annual number of new HIV infections by 25%

Objective 2*
By 2015, increase the percentage of people living with HIV who know their serostatus to 90%

Objective 3
By 2015, increase the percentage of people diagnosed with HIV infection at earlier stages of disease (not stage 3: AIDS), by 25%

Objective 4
By 2015, decrease the rate of perinatally acquired pediatric HIV cases by 25%

Objective 5
By 2015, reduce the proportion of MSM who reported unprotected anal intercourse during their last sexual encounter with a partner of discordant or unknown HIV status by 25%

Objective 6
By 2015, reduce the proportion of IDU who reported risky sexual or drug using behavior by 25%

Strategy A1
Systematically collect, analyze, integrate, and disseminate data to monitor the HIV epidemic, assess the impact of HIV prevention activities, and guide the national response

Strategy A2
Identify drivers of HIV incidence in priority populations (as identified in NHAS) to design and target effective interventions and strategies for maximum impact

Strategy A3
Identify, develop and evaluate effective behavioral, biomedical and structural technologies, interventions and strategies; prioritize this process to maximize reduction of HIV acquisition among high-incidence populations

Strategy A4
Implement and evaluate effective behavioral, structural, and biomedical technologies, interventions and strategies at scale; prioritize and target implementation to maximally reduce HIV acquisition in high-incidence populations

*Objective taken from NHAS

GOAL B: PREVENTION AND CARE—Increase Linkage to and Impact of Prevention and Care Services with People Living with HIV/AIDS

Objective 1*
By 2015, reduce the HIV transmission rate by 30%

Objective 2*
By 2015, increase the percentage of persons diagnosed with HIV who are linked to clinical care as evidenced by having a CD4 count or viral load measure within 3 months of HIV diagnosis to 85%

Objective 3
By 2015, increase by 10% the percentage of HIV-diagnosed persons in care whose most recent viral load test in the past 12 months was undetectable

Objective 4
By 2015, reduce the percentage of HIV-diagnosed persons in care who report unprotected anal or vaginal intercourse during the last 12 months with partners of discordant or unknown HIV status by 33%

Strategy B1
Identify, develop, and evaluate interventions, strategies, and technologies to increase linkage to care and use of ART; maximize adherence to ART and retention in care; reduce transmission risk behaviors; and provide partner services

Strategy B2
Ensure the implementation and evaluation of interventions, strategies, and technologies to increase linkage to care and use of ART; maximize adherence to ART and retention in care; reduce transmission risk behaviors; and provide partner services

*Objective taken from NHAS

GOAL C: HEALTH DISPARITIES—Reduce HIV-Related Disparities

Objective 1*
By 2015, increase the percentage of HIV-diagnosed MSM with undetectable viral load by 20%

Objective 2*
By 2015, increase the percentage of HIV-diagnosed Blacks with undetectable viral load by 20%

Objective 3*
By 2015, increase the percentage of HIV-diagnosed Hispanics with undetectable viral load by 20%

Objective 4
By 2015, reduce the annual number of new HIV infections among MSM, Blacks, Hispanics and IDU by at least 25% in each group

Objective 5
By 2015, ensure the percentage of persons diagnosed with HIV who have a CD4 count within 3 months of HIV diagnosis is 75% or greater for all racial/ethnic groups

Strategy C1
Target resources and activities to reduce HIV-related disparities (through Goals A and B)

Strategy C2
Monitor national trends and DHAP activities and outcomes to ensure that HIV-related disparities and their underlying factors are reduced (through Goals A and B)

Strategy C3
Communicate DHAP activities and progress to stakeholders and enlist partners to advance activities that reduce disparities (to be coordinated with Strategy D2 partnership engagement framework)

Strategy C4
Ensure the cultural and linguistic appropriateness of DHAP activities and materials to increase their impact

*Objective taken from NHAS

GOAL D: ORGANIZATIONAL EXCELLENCE—
Promote a Skilled and Engaged Workforce and Effective, Efficient Operations to Ensure the Successful Delivery of CDC's HIV Prevention Science, Programs and Policies

Objective 1
Each year, all branches and operating units will complete at least 80% of their work plan activities

Objective 2
Each year, all branches and operating units will adhere to 80% of their administrative and extramural processing deadlines

Objective
By 2015, DHAP will have improved its rating on the HHS Annual Employee Viewpoint Survey

Strategy D1
Develop, implement and monitor an internal communication plan with two-way communication channels to improve transparency, accountability, participation and coordination both within DHAP and with other CDC stakeholders

Strategy D2
Develop, implement and monitor an external communication and partner engagement plan to improve transparency, accountability, participation and collaboration through bi-directional flow of information

Strategy D3
Maximize the effectiveness of DHAP human and financial resources to achieve DHAP's strategic goals and objectives

Strategy D4
Allocate extramural resources and use results-oriented management to improve accountability and maximize the impact of all DHAP-supported activities on the HIV epidemic

Appendix C — Links to NHAS and NCHHSTP Plans

DHAP Strategic Plan 2011-2015 Goals and Strategy Alignment with the *National HIV/AIDS Strategy for the United States (NHAS) Implementation Plan* and the *National Center for HIV/AIDS, Viral Hepatitis, STD, and TB Prevention Strategic Plan, 2010-2015*

DHAP GOAL A: HIV Incidence—Prevent New Infections		
DHAP Strategy	**Linked National HIV/AIDS Strategy Implementation Plan Step(s)[1]**	**Linked NCHHSTP Strategic Plan Objective(s)[2]**
A1: Systematically collect, analyze, integrate, and disseminate data to monitor the HIV epidemic, assess the impact of HIV prevention activities, and guide the national response	Goal: Reducing HIV-Related Health Disparities; Step 2.2 Measure and utilize community viral load	Goal 2: Program Collaboration and Service Integration (PCSI); Objective 2B. Align surveillance systems, policies, standards, and procedures so that surveillance data can be accessed and used for integrated public health interventions, integrated programmatic planning, and evaluation
A2: Identify drivers of HIV incidence in priority populations (as identified in the NHAS) to design and target effective interventions and strategies for maximum impact	Goal: Reducing New HIV Infections; Step 1.2 Target high risk populations	Goal 3. Health Equity; Objective 3C. Identify which social determinants of health are important to address to reduce health disparities in HIV/AIDS, viral hepatitis, STDs, and TB and develop and advance appropriate plans for addressing these social determinants in NCHHSTP programmatic and scientific work
A3: Identify, develop and evaluate effective behavioral, biomedical and structural technologies, interventions and strategies; prioritize this process to maximize reduction of HIV acquisition among high-incidence populations	Goal: Reducing New HIV Infections; Step 2.1 Design and evaluate innovative prevention strategies and combination approaches for preventing HIV in high risk communities Goal: Reducing HIV-Related Health Disparities; Step 2.3 Promote a more holistic approach to health	Goal 1: Prevention Through Healthcare; Objective 1D. Promote innovative, systems- and health-based approaches to the prevention and control of HIV, viral hepatitis, STDs, and TB Goal 2: Program Collaboration and Service Integration (PCSI); Objective 2E. Conduct research and evaluation related to PCSI
A4: Implement and evaluate effective behavioral, structural, and biomedical technologies, interventions and strategies at scale; prioritize and target implementation to maximally reduce HIV acquisition in high-incidence populations	Goal: Reducing New HIV Infections; Step 1.2.1 Prevent HIV among gay and bisexual men and transgender individuals Goal: Reducing New HIV Infections; Step 1.2.2 Prevent HIV among Black men and women Goal: Reducing New HIV Infections; Step 1.2.3 Prevent HIV among Latinos and Latinas Goal: Reducing New HIV Infections; Step 1.2.4 Prevent HIV among substance users Goal: Reducing New HIV Infections; Step 1.3 Address HIV prevention in Asian American and Pacific Islander and American Indian and Alaska Native populations Goal: Reducing New HIV Infections; Step 2.3 Expand access to effective prevention services Goal: Reducing New HIV Infections; Step 3.1 Utilize social marketing and education campaigns Goal: Reducing HIV-Related Health Disparities; Step 2.3 Promote a more holistic approach to health	Goal 2: Program Collaboration and Service Integration (PCSI); Objective 2A. Expand programmatic flexibility to facilitate program collaboration and the integration of services at the client level Goal 2: Program Collaboration and Service Integration (PCSI); Objective 2C. Identify and promote opportunities for integrated trainings, cross-training, and training on integration for NCHHSTP and jurisdictions Goal 2: Program Collaboration and Service Integration (PCSI); Objective 2D. Implement, maintain, and evaluate support systems, policies, structures, and activities designed to enhance PCSI

[1] Table links only those steps in the National HIV/AIDS Strategy Federal Implementation Plan for which CDC is listed as either a Lead Agency or Other Agency.

[2] Table does not include objectives from NCHHSTP Goal 4 Global Health Protection and Health Systems Strengthening.

DHAP GOAL B: Prevention and Care—Increase Linkage to and Impact of Prevention and Care Services with People Living with HIV/AIDS		
DHAP Strategy	**Linked National HIV/AIDS Strategy Implementation Plan Step(s)[1]**	**Linked NCHHSTP Strategic Plan Objective(s)[2]**
B1: Identify, develop, and evaluate interventions, strategies, and technologies to increase linkage to care and use of ART; maximize adherence to ART and retention in care; reduce transmission risk behaviors; and provide partner services	Goal: Reducing New HIV Infections; Step 2.1 Design and evaluate innovative prevention strategies and combination approaches for preventing HIV in high risk communities Goal: Reducing New HIV Infections; Step 2.4 Expand prevention with HIV-positive individuals Goal: Reducing HIV-Related Health Disparities; Step 2.3 Promote a more holistic approach to health	Goal 1: Prevention Through Healthcare; Objective 1B. Maximize opportunities to advance NCHHSTP strategic priorities in a transformed health system
B2: Ensure the implementation and evaluation of interventions, strategies, and technologies to increase linkage to care and use of ART; maximize adherence to ART and retention in care; reduce transmission risk behaviors; and provide partner services	Goal: Reducing New HIV Infections; Step 2.4 Expand prevention with HIV-positive individuals Goal: Increasing Access to Care and Improving Health Outcomes for People Living with HIV; Step 1.1 Facilitate linkages to care Goal: Increasing Access to Care and Improving Health Outcomes for People Living with HIV; Step 1.2 Promote collaboration among providers Goal: Increasing Access to Care and Improving Health Outcomes for People Living with HIV; Step 1.3 Maintain people living with HIV in care Goal: Reducing HIV-Related Health Disparities; Step 1.1 Ensure that high risk groups have access to regular viral load and CD4 tests Goal: Reducing HIV-Related Health Disparities; Step 2.3 Promote a more holistic approach to health	Goal 1: Prevention Through Healthcare; Objective 1C. Monitor performance and quality of prevention services and interventions

[1] Table links only those steps in the National HIV/AIDS Strategy Federal Implementation Plan for which CDC is listed as either a Lead Agency or Other Agency.
[2] Table does not include objectives from NCHHSTP Goal 4 Global Health Protection and Health Systems Strengthening.

DHAP GOAL C: Health Disparities—Reduce HIV-Related Disparities

DHAP Strategy	Linked National HIV/AIDS Strategy Implementation Plan Step(s)[1]	Linked NCHHSTP Strategic Plan Objective(s)[2]
C1: Target resources and activities to reduce HIV-related disparities (through Goals A and B)	Goal: Reducing New HIV Infections; Step 1.1 Allocate public funding to geographic areas consistent with the epidemic Goal: Reducing New HIV Infections; Step 1.2 Target high risk populations	Goal 3. Health Equity; Objective 3A. Define and pursue a science-based approach to identify and eliminate health disparities related to HIV/AIDS, viral hepatitis, STDs, and TB and associated diseases and conditions
C2: Monitor national trends and DHAP activities and outcomes to ensure that HIV-related disparities and their underlying factors are reduced (through Goals A and B)	Goal: Reducing HIV-Related Health Disparities; Step 2.2 Measure and utilize community viral load	Goal 3. Health Equity; Objective 3C. Indentify which social determinants of health are important to address to reduce health disparities in HIV/AIDS, viral hepatitis, STDs, and TB and develop and advance appropriate plans for addressing these social determinants in NCHHSTP programmatic and scientific work
C3: Communicate DHAP activities and progress to stakeholders and enlist partners to advance activities that reduce disparities (to be coordinated with Strategy D2 partnership engagement framework)	Goal: Reducing HIV-Related Health Disparities; Step 3.2 Promote public leadership of people living with HIV Goal: Reducing HIV-Related Health Disparities; Step 2.3 Promote a more holistic approach to health	Goal 3. Health Equity; Objective 3B. Mobilize partners and stakeholders to promote health equity and social determinants of health as it relates to HIV, viral hepatitis, STD, and TB prevention
C4: Ensure the cultural and linguistic appropriateness of DHAP activities and materials to increase their impact	NONE LINKED	Goal 3. Health Equity; Objective 3B. Mobilize partners and stakeholders to promote health equity and social determinants of health as it relates to HIV, viral hepatitis, STD, and TB prevention

[1] Table links only those steps in the National HIV/AIDS Strategy Federal Implementation Plan for which CDC is listed as either a Lead Agency or Other Agency.
[2] Table does not include objectives from NCHHSTP Goal 4 Global Health Protection and Health Systems Strengthening.

DHAP GOAL D: Organizational Excellence—Promote a Skilled and Engaged Workforce and Effective, Efficient Operations to Ensure the Successful Delivery of CDC's HIV Prevention Science, Programs and Policies

DHAP Strategy	Linked National HIV/AIDS Strategy Implementation Plan Step(s)[1]	Linked NCHHSTP Strategic Plan Objective(s)[2]
D1: Develop, implement and monitor an internal communication plan with two-way communication channels to improve transparency, accountability, participation and coordination both within DHAP and with other CDC stakeholders	Goal: Reducing HIV-Related Health Disparities; Step 2.3 Promote a more holistic approach to health	NONE LINKED
D2: Develop, implement and monitor an external communication and partner engagement plan to improve transparency, accountability, participation and collaboration through bi-directional flow of information	Goal: Reducing New HIV Infections; Step 3.2 Promote age-appropriate HIV and STI prevention education for all Americans Goal: Reducing HIV-Related Health Disparities; Step 2.3 Promote a more holistic approach to health	Goal 1: Prevention Through Healthcare; Objective 1A. Maximize opportunities to adopt, integrate and leverage NCHHSTP prevention priorities into other HHS Operational Divisions and other federal agencies Goal 5. Partnerships; Objective 5A. Increase the partnership capacity of NCHHSTP by supporting and facilitating partnership outreach and communication to existing and new partners Goal 5. Partnerships; Objective 5B. Increase understanding of and support for NCHHSTP's mission, research, programs, and policies among network partners Goal 5. Partnerships; Objective 5C. Increase the collaborative partnership capacity of NCHHSTP by using multi-level real-time communication technologies and other mechanisms to meet the increased communication needs of collaborative partners Goal 5. Partnerships; Objective 5D. Coordinate NCHHSTP partnership and program activities with and among CDC centers and offices, federal agencies, non-profit, and private sector entities to increase collaborative efforts and to enhance the efficiency, implementation, and dissemination of programs and information
D3: Maximize the effectiveness of DHAP human and financial resources to achieve DHAP's strategic goals and objectives	Goal: Reducing New HIV Infections; Step 1.1 Allocate public funding to geographic areas consistent with the epidemic	Goal 6: Workforce Development; Objective 6A. Attract, recruit, and retain a prepared, diverse, and sustainable workforce to address all NCHHSTP diseases and conditions Goal 6: Workforce Development; Objective 6B. Continuously provide staff with development opportunities to ensure the effective and innovative delivery of NCHHSTP programs Goal 6: Workforce Development; Objective 6C. Continuously recognize performance, contributions, and achievements of employees and create an atmosphere that promotes a healthy work-life balance
D4: Allocate extramural resources and use results-oriented management to improve accountability and maximize the impact of all DHAP-supported activities on the HIV epidemic	Goal: Reducing New HIV Infections; Step 1.1 Allocate public funding to geographic areas consistent with the epidemic Goal: Reducing New HIV Infections; Step 1.4 Enhance program accountability Goal: Achieving a More Coordinated National Response; Step 2.3 Encourage states to provide regular progress reports	NONE LINKED

[1] Table links only those steps in the National HIV/AIDS Strategy Federal Implementation Plan for which CDC is listed as either a Lead Agency or Other Agency.
[2] Table does not include objectives from NCHHSTP Goal 4 Global Health Protection and Health Systems Strengthening.

Appendix D — Goals and Objectives with Baselines, Targets, and Data Source

DHAP GOAL A: HIV Incidence—Prevent New Infections		
DHAP Objective	**Baseline & Target**	**Data Source**
Goal A, Objective 1: By 2015, reduce the annual number of new HIV infections by 25%*	Baseline: 2006 - 56,300 Target: 2015 - 42,225	HIV Surveillance, HIV incidence surveillance
Goal A, Objective 2: By 2015, increase the percentage of people living with HIV who know their serostatus to 90%*	Baseline: 2006 - 79% Target: 2015 - 90%	HIV Surveillance, statistical estimation methods
Goal A, Objective 3: By 2015, increase the percentage of people diagnosed with HIV infection at earlier stages of disease (not stage 3: AIDS), by 25%	Baseline: 42.5% Target: 2015 – 53.1%	HIV Surveillance
Goal A, Objective 4: By 2015, decrease the rate of perinatally acquired pediatric HIV cases by 25%	Baseline: 2008 - 0.9 per 100,000 infants Target: 2015 - 0.7 per 100,000 infants	HIV Surveillance
Goal A, Objective 5: By 2015, reduce the proportion of MSM who reported unprotected anal intercourse during their last sexual encounter with a partner of discordant or unknown HIV status by 25%	Baseline: 2008 - 13.5% Target: 2015 - 10.1%	National HIV Behavioral Surveillance System
Goal A, Objective 6: By 2015, reduce the proportion of IDU who reported risky sexual or drug using behavior by 25%	Baseline: 2009 - 73% Target: 2015 - 55%	National HIV Behavioral Surveillance System

*Objective taken from NHAS

DHAP GOAL B: Prevention and Care—Increase Linkage to and Impact of Prevention and Care Services with People Living with HIV/AIDS

DHAP Objective	Baseline & Target	Data Source
Goal B, Objective 1: By 2015, reduce the HIV transmission rate by 30%*	Baseline: 2006 - 5.0 per 100 persons living with HIV Target: 2015 - 3.5 per 100 persons living with HIV	Calculations of HIV incidence and prevalence, utilizing the HIV incidence surveillance and national prevalence estimates
Goal B, Objective 2: By 2015, increase the percentage of persons diagnosed with HIV who are linked to clinical care as evidenced by having a CD4 count or viral load measure within 3 months of HIV diagnosis to 85%*	Baseline: 2007 – 60% Target: 2015 – 85%	HIV Surveillance
Goal B, Objective 3: By 2015, increase by 10% the percentage of HIV-diagnosed persons in care whose most recent viral load test in the past 12 months was undetectable	Baseline: 2009 – data to be available 9/2011 Target: 2015 - pending	Medical Monitoring Project
Goal B, Objective 4: By 2015, reduce the percentage of HIV-diagnosed persons in care who report unprotected anal or vaginal intercourse during the last 12 months with partners of discordant or unknown HIV status by 33%	Baseline: 2009 – data to be available 9/2011 Target: 2015 – pending	Medical Monitoring Project

*Objective taken from NHAS

DHAP GOAL C: Health Disparities—Reduce HIV-Related Disparities		
DHAP Strategy	**Baseline & Target**	**Data Source**
Goal C, Objective 1: By 2015, increase the percentage of HIV-diagnosed MSM with undetectable viral load by 20%*	Baseline: 2008 - data to be available 8/2011 Target: 2015 - pending	HIV Surveillance
Goal C, Objective 2: By 2015, increase the percentage of HIV-diagnosed Blacks with undetectable viral load by 20%*	Baseline: 2008 - data to be available 8/2011 Target: 2015 - pending	HIV Surveillance
Goal C, Objective 3: By 2015, increase the percentage of HIV-diagnosed Hispanics with undetectable viral load by 20%*	Baseline: 2008 – data to be available 8/2011 Target: 2015 - pending	HIV Surveillance
Goal C, Objective 4: By 2015, reduce the annual number of new HIV infections among MSM, Blacks, Hispanics and IDU by at least 25% in each group	Baseline (all 2006): MSM: 30,800 Blacks: 24,900 Hispanics: 9,700 IDU: 6,600 Targets (all 2015): MSM: 23,100 Blacks: 18,675 Hispanics: 7275 IDU: 4950 Note: MSM includes MSM/IDU	HIV Surveillance
Goal C, Objective 5: By 2015, ensure the percentage of persons diagnosed with HIV who have a CD4 count within 3 months of HIV diagnosis is 75% or greater for all racial/ethnic groups	Baseline: 2007- data to be available 8/2011 Target: 2015 - pending	HIV Surveillance

*Objective taken from NHAS

DHAP GOAL D: Organizational Excellence— Promote a Skilled and Engaged Workforce and Effective, Efficient Operations to Ensure the Successful Delivery of CDC's HIV Prevention Science, Programs and Policies

DHAP Strategy	Baseline & Target	Data Source
Goal D, Objective 1: Each year, all branches and operating units will complete at least 80% of their work plan activities	Baseline: Not applicable Targets: 2015 – 80%	Internal Branch/Operating Unit Work Plan Tracking Database
Goal D, Objective 2: Each year, all branches and operating units will adhere to 80% of their administrative and extramural processing deadlines	Baseline: Not applicable Targets: FY2011 – 80%	Internal Administrative Processes Tracking Database
Goal D, Objective 3: By 2015, DHAP will have improved its rating on the HHS Annual Employee Viewpoint Survey	Baseline: Pending Target: 2015 – Pending	HHS Annual Employee Viewpoint Survey

*Objective taken from NHAS

Notes

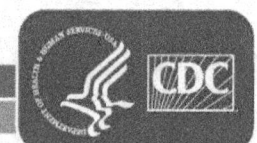